HOW TO BOOST YOUR FERTILITY NATURALLY

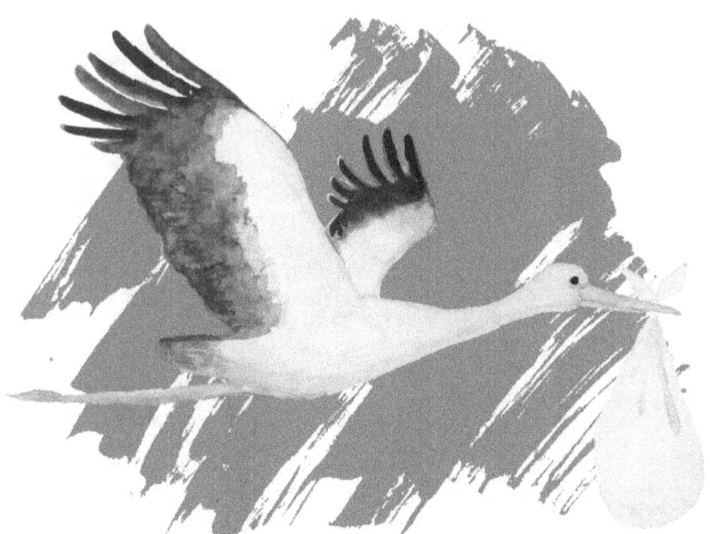

Aurora Brooks

xspurts.com

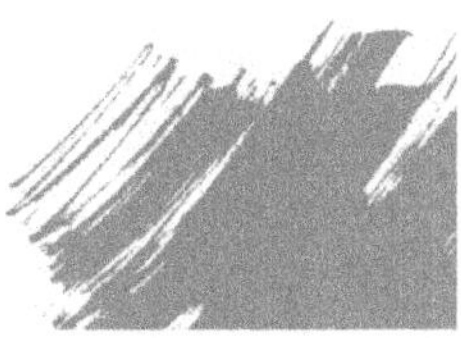

Free Book Offer:
Get How to be a Super Mom For Free

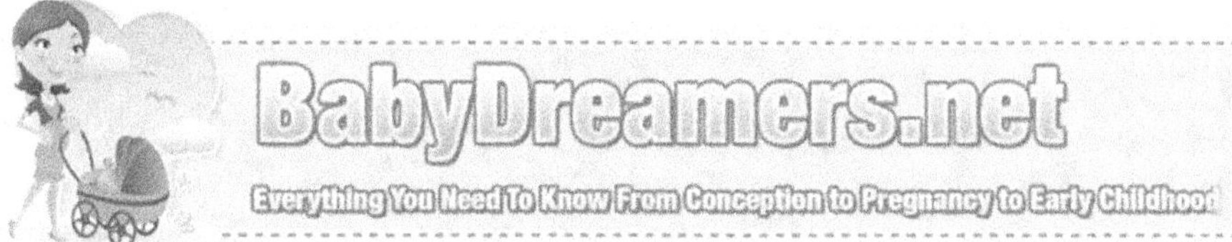

A Short Read is a type of book that is designed to be read in one quick sitting.

These no fluff books are perfect for people who want an overview about a subject in a short period of time.

Table of Contents

CONSIDER HERBAL SUPPLEMENTS

CONSULT WITH A HEALTHCARE PROFESSIONAL

HAVE REGULAR SEXUAL INTERCOURSE

TIMING INTERCOURSE WITH OVULATION

ENJOY THE PROCESS

FREQUENTLY ASKED QUESTIONS

Have Questions / Comments?

Get How To Be A Super Mom 100% FREE

How to Boost Your Fertility Naturally

Are you looking for ways to boost your fertility without medical intervention? Look no further! In this article, we will explore various tips and techniques that can naturally increase your chances of conceiving. By making simple lifestyle changes and adopting healthy habits, you can optimize your fertility and increase your chances of starting or expanding your family.

Eat a Healthy Diet

When it comes to boosting fertility naturally, one of the most important factors to consider is your diet. The food you consume plays a significant role in your reproductive health and can have a direct impact on your fertility. By making smart choices and incorporating certain foods into your diet, you can increase your chances of conceiving.

A healthy diet for fertility should include a variety of nutrient-rich foods that support reproductive function. This means focusing on whole, unprocessed foods that are packed with vitamins, minerals, and antioxidants. Some key nutrients to prioritize include folate, iron, zinc, and vitamins C and E.

To ensure you're getting these essential nutrients, include plenty of fruits and vegetables in your diet. These colorful foods are not only rich in antioxidants but also provide important vitamins and minerals. Additionally, opt for whole grains, lean proteins, and healthy fats such as avocados and nuts.

It's also important to stay hydrated by drinking plenty of water throughout the day. Proper hydration supports overall health and can help maintain optimal reproductive function. Aim to drink at least eight glasses of water daily.

While there are no specific foods that guarantee fertility, certain options have been associated with improved reproductive health. For instance, research suggests that consuming more omega-3 fatty acids, found in fatty fish like salmon, may enhance fertility. Similarly, incorporating foods high in antioxidants, such as berries and leafy greens, can help protect your eggs and sperm from damage.

Remember, a healthy diet is just one piece of the puzzle when it comes to boosting fertility naturally. It's important to combine it with other lifestyle changes and strategies for optimal results. By nourishing your body with the right foods, you can support your reproductive system and increase your chances of conceiving.

Manage Stress Levels

Stress can have a significant impact on fertility. When we experience high levels of stress, our bodies release cortisol, a hormone that can interfere with reproductive hormones and disrupt the delicate balance needed for conception. It's important to recognize the connection between stress and fertility and take steps to manage stress levels.

There are several strategies for stress reduction that can help improve fertility. One effective approach is practicing mindfulness. Mindfulness involves being present in the moment and focusing on your thoughts and sensations without judgment. This can help reduce stress and promote a sense of calm and relaxation. Consider incorporating mindfulness techniques such as meditation or deep breathing exercises into your daily routine.

Engaging in relaxation techniques can also be beneficial for managing stress and enhancing fertility. These techniques can include activities such as yoga, tai chi, or progressive muscle relaxation. These practices help release tension from the body and promote a state of relaxation. By regularly incorporating relaxation techniques into your routine, you can reduce stress and create a more favorable environment for conception.

In addition to these techniques, it's important to prioritize self-care and engage in activities that bring you joy and relaxation. This can include hobbies, spending time in nature, or connecting with loved ones. Taking time for yourself and finding healthy outlets for stress can significantly improve your overall well-being and fertility.

Practice Mindfulness

Mindfulness is a powerful practice that can significantly reduce stress levels and improve fertility. By being fully present in the moment and cultivating a non-judgmental awareness of our thoughts, feelings, and sensations, mindfulness helps to calm the mind and relax the body. This, in turn, reduces the production of stress hormones, such as cortisol, which can have a negative impact on fertility.

When we are stressed, our body goes into "fight or flight" mode, diverting resources away from non-essential functions like reproduction. By practicing mindfulness, we can activate the body's relaxation response, allowing it to focus on reproductive processes and increasing the chances of conception.

There are various techniques you can incorporate into your daily routine to practice mindfulness. One effective method is deep breathing exercises. By taking slow, deep breaths and focusing on the sensation of the breath entering and leaving your body, you can bring yourself into the present moment and alleviate stress.

Another mindfulness technique is body scanning. This involves systematically directing your attention to different parts of your body, noticing any sensations or tensions, and consciously releasing any areas of tension. Body scanning helps to promote relaxation and awareness of the body, enhancing fertility.

Additionally, meditation is a powerful mindfulness practice that can be beneficial for reducing stress and improving fertility. By setting aside a few minutes each day to sit quietly and focus your attention on your breath or a specific object, you can cultivate a sense of calm and balance in your life.

Incorporating mindfulness into your daily routine can have a profound impact on your overall well-being and fertility. By reducing stress levels and promoting relaxation, mindfulness can create a more fertile environment within your body, increasing the likelihood of conception.

Engage in Relaxation Techniques

Engaging in relaxation techniques can be a powerful tool in promoting fertility. When it comes to conceiving, stress and anxiety can have a significant impact on your reproductive health. By incorporating relaxation techniques into your daily routine, you can reduce stress levels and increase your chances of getting pregnant.

There are various relaxation techniques that you can try, each offering its own unique benefits. Here are a few techniques that can help promote fertility:

- **Meditation:** Meditation is a practice that involves focusing your mind and eliminating the stream of thoughts that may be causing stress. By taking a few minutes each day to meditate, you can calm your mind, reduce stress, and create a positive environment for conception.
- **Deep Breathing:** Deep breathing exercises are a simple yet effective way to relax your body and mind. By taking slow, deep breaths and focusing on your breath, you can activate your body's relaxation response and reduce stress hormones.
- **Progressive Muscle Relaxation:** Progressive muscle relaxation involves systematically tensing and then relaxing each muscle group in your body. This technique helps release tension and promotes a state of deep relaxation.

- **Yoga:** Yoga combines physical postures, breathing exercises, and meditation to promote physical and mental well-being. Practicing yoga regularly can improve blood flow to the reproductive organs, reduce stress, and balance hormones.
- **Aromatherapy:** Aromatherapy involves using essential oils to promote relaxation and reduce stress. Certain scents, such as lavender and chamomile, have been shown to have calming effects and can be used during relaxation exercises.

Remember, finding the right relaxation technique for you may take some trial and error. It's important to listen to your body and choose techniques that resonate with you. By incorporating relaxation techniques into your daily routine, you can create a calm and nurturing environment for conception.

Exercise Regularly

Exercise plays a crucial role in boosting fertility and improving reproductive health. Regular physical activity not only helps maintain a healthy weight but also has numerous benefits for fertility. Here are some of the key advantages of exercising for fertility:

- **Enhances Hormonal Balance:** Engaging in regular exercise helps regulate hormone levels in the body, including reproductive hormones. This can improve the overall functioning of the reproductive system and increase the chances of conception.
- **Improves Blood Circulation:** Exercise promotes better blood flow throughout the body, including the reproductive organs. This increased circulation can enhance the delivery of oxygen and nutrients to the reproductive system, supporting optimal fertility.
- **Reduces Insulin Resistance:** Regular physical activity can help reduce insulin resistance, a condition that can interfere with ovulation and fertility. By improving insulin sensitivity, exercise can enhance reproductive function.
- **Manages Stress:** Exercise is a fantastic stress-reliever and can help manage stress levels, which can have a significant impact on fertility. By reducing stress, exercise creates a more favorable environment for conception.

When it comes to the types of physical activity recommended for fertility, it's important to find a balance. Here are some exercises that are beneficial for fertility:

- **Cardiovascular Exercises:** Activities like brisk walking, jogging, swimming, and cycling are excellent choices for improving cardiovascular health and promoting fertility.

- **Strength Training:** Incorporating strength training exercises, such as weightlifting or resistance training, can help build muscle mass and improve overall fitness, which can positively impact fertility.
- **Yoga or Pilates:** These mind-body exercises not only provide physical benefits but also help reduce stress and promote relaxation. Yoga and Pilates can enhance fertility by improving blood flow to the reproductive organs and reducing tension in the body.

Remember, it's important to consult with a healthcare professional or fertility specialist before starting any new exercise routine, especially if you have any underlying medical conditions or concerns. They can provide personalized recommendations based on your specific needs and goals.

Aim for Moderate Exercise

Aim for Moderate Exercise

When it comes to boosting fertility, exercise plays a crucial role. However, it's important to find the right balance. While intense workouts may seem like the best way to get in shape, they can actually have a negative impact on fertility. Instead, aiming for moderate exercise can be more beneficial for your reproductive health.

Intense workouts can put excessive stress on your body, leading to hormonal imbalances that can interfere with ovulation and menstrual regularity. On the other hand, moderate exercise helps to regulate hormones and improve blood flow to the reproductive organs, creating a more conducive environment for conception.

So, what constitutes moderate exercise? It can vary from person to person, but generally, it means engaging in activities that get your heart rate up and make you break a sweat, but still allow you to carry on a conversation without feeling completely out of breath. Examples include brisk walking, cycling, swimming, and dancing.

Incorporating moderate exercise into your routine not only enhances your fertility, but it also has numerous other benefits for your overall well-being. It can help manage weight, reduce stress, improve mood, and increase energy levels. Remember, the goal is to find a balance that supports your reproductive health without overexerting yourself.

Include Yoga or Pilates

Yoga and Pilates are two popular forms of exercise that can have a positive impact on fertility and reproductive health. Both practices focus on strengthening the body, improving flexibility, and promoting overall well-being. By incorporating yoga or Pilates into your routine, you can enhance your fertility journey and improve your chances of conception.

Yoga, an ancient practice originating from India, combines physical postures, breathing exercises, and meditation. It is known for its ability to reduce stress, increase blood flow to the reproductive organs, and balance hormone levels. Certain yoga poses, such as the butterfly pose and the legs-up-the-wall pose, specifically target the pelvic area and can help improve circulation and stimulate the reproductive organs.

Pilates, on the other hand, is a low-impact exercise method that focuses on core strength, flexibility, and body alignment. By strengthening the core muscles, Pilates can improve posture and support the reproductive organs. Additionally, Pilates exercises can help increase blood flow to the pelvic area and improve overall muscle tone.

Both yoga and Pilates provide an opportunity to connect with your body and reduce stress, which is crucial for optimizing fertility. Engaging in these practices can help regulate menstrual cycles, improve hormonal balance, and create a nurturing environment for conception.

If you're new to yoga or Pilates, it's recommended to start with beginner-friendly classes or seek guidance from a certified instructor. They can help you learn proper techniques and modify exercises based on your individual needs. Remember to listen to your body and take it at your own pace.

Incorporating yoga or Pilates into your fertility journey not only benefits your physical health but also promotes emotional well-being. It allows you to take time for yourself, relax, and focus on the present moment. So, why not give yoga or Pilates a try and enhance your fertility naturally?

Maintain a Healthy Weight

Maintain a Healthy Weight

Weight plays a crucial role in fertility, as both being underweight or overweight can have negative effects on reproductive health. It is important to achieve and maintain a healthy weight to optimize your chances of conceiving. Excess body fat can disrupt hormonal balance and interfere with ovulation, while being underweight can lead to irregular or absent menstrual cycles.

To achieve a healthy weight, it is essential to focus on a balanced diet and regular exercise. Here are some tips to help you maintain a healthy weight:

- Eat a nutritious diet: Include plenty of fruits, vegetables, whole grains, lean proteins, and healthy fats in your meals. Avoid processed foods, sugary snacks, and excessive consumption of refined carbohydrates.
- Portion control: Pay attention to portion sizes and avoid overeating. Use smaller plates and bowls to help control your portions.
- Stay hydrated: Drink an adequate amount of water throughout the day to support your metabolism and maintain a healthy weight.
- Engage in regular physical activity: Aim for at least 30 minutes of moderate-intensity exercise most days of the week. Choose activities that you enjoy, such as brisk walking, swimming, or cycling.
- Seek professional guidance: If you are struggling with weight management, consider consulting a registered dietitian or a healthcare professional who can provide personalized guidance and support.

Remember, achieving a healthy weight is a gradual process, and it is important to be patient with yourself. Focus on making sustainable lifestyle changes rather than resorting to crash diets or extreme exercise regimens. By maintaining a healthy weight, you can improve your fertility and increase your chances of conceiving.

Avoid Extreme Weight Loss

Extreme weight loss can have a detrimental impact on fertility and disrupt the delicate balance of reproductive hormones. When the body experiences rapid weight loss, it can trigger hormonal imbalances that interfere with ovulation and the menstrual cycle. This can make it more difficult for women to conceive and increase the risk of irregular periods or even amenorrhea, the absence of menstruation.

Additionally, extreme weight loss can lead to a decrease in estrogen production, which is crucial for maintaining a healthy reproductive system. Estrogen plays a vital role in regulating the menstrual cycle and promoting the growth and development of the uterine lining, necessary for the implantation of a fertilized egg. Insufficient estrogen levels can hinder the chances of successful conception.

Furthermore, extreme weight loss can also affect the production of other reproductive hormones, such as progesterone. Progesterone is essential for preparing the uterus for implantation and supporting early pregnancy. Insufficient levels of progesterone can result in a shortened luteal phase, making it challenging for a fertilized egg to implant and sustain a pregnancy.

It is important to note that maintaining a healthy weight is crucial for fertility, but extreme weight loss should be avoided. If you are planning to conceive, it is recommended to consult with a healthcare professional or a registered dietitian who specializes in fertility to ensure that you are following a balanced and nutritious diet that supports your reproductive health without resorting to extreme measures.

Address Obesity

Addressing obesity is crucial for improving fertility as there is a strong relationship between obesity and reproductive health. Excess weight can disrupt hormonal balance, leading to irregular menstrual cycles and ovulation problems. It can also increase the risk of conditions such as polycystic ovary syndrome (PCOS), which can further impact fertility.

To address weight concerns and enhance fertility, it is important to adopt healthy lifestyle habits. Here are some steps you can take:

- 1. Follow a balanced diet: Focus on consuming nutrient-dense foods such as fruits, vegetables, whole grains, and lean proteins. Avoid processed foods, sugary snacks, and beverages.
- 2. Control portion sizes: Be mindful of portion sizes to prevent overeating. Use smaller plates and bowls to help manage portions.
- 3. Engage in regular physical activity: Incorporate regular exercise into your routine. Aim for at least 150 minutes of moderate-intensity aerobic activity per week, such as brisk walking or swimming.
- 4. Seek professional guidance: Consult with a healthcare professional or a registered dietitian to create a personalized weight loss plan that suits your needs.
- 5. Set realistic goals: Gradual and sustainable weight loss is key. Aim to lose 1-2 pounds per week, as rapid weight loss can negatively impact fertility.

By addressing obesity and achieving a healthy weight, you can improve your chances of conceiving and enhance overall reproductive health. Remember, it's important to consult with healthcare professionals for personalized guidance and support throughout your weight loss journey.

Get Sufficient Sleep

Sleep plays a crucial role in maintaining overall health and well-being, and it is no different when it comes to fertility. Getting sufficient sleep is essential for optimizing fertility and increasing the chances of conception. Adequate rest allows the body to regulate hormones, including those involved in the reproductive system. Lack of sleep can disrupt hormone levels, leading to irregular menstrual cycles and decreased fertility.

To improve sleep quality and promote fertility, here are some tips to consider:

- **Establish a Bedtime Routine:** Creating a consistent bedtime routine can signal to your body that it's time to wind down and prepare for sleep. This can include activities such as reading a book, taking a warm bath, or practicing relaxation techniques.
- **Avoid Electronic Devices Before Bed:** The blue light emitted by electronic devices like smartphones, tablets, and laptops can interfere with the production of melatonin, a hormone that regulates sleep. Minimize exposure to screens at least an hour before bed to improve sleep quality.

By prioritizing sleep and implementing these tips, you can support your fertility journey and increase the likelihood of conceiving.

Establish a Bedtime Routine

Establishing a bedtime routine is essential for promoting better sleep and fertility. A relaxing routine before bed can help calm the mind and prepare the body for restful sleep, which is crucial for reproductive health. Here are some tips to help you create a bedtime routine that promotes better sleep and fertility:

- **Create a Consistent Schedule:** Go to bed and wake up at the same time every day, even on weekends. This helps regulate your body's internal clock and promotes better sleep quality.
- **Avoid Stimulants:** Stay away from caffeine, nicotine, and alcohol in the evening, as they can interfere with your ability to fall asleep and stay asleep.
- **Unwind with Relaxation Techniques:** Engage in activities that help you relax and unwind before bed. This can include reading a book, taking a warm bath, practicing deep breathing exercises, or listening to calming music.
- **Create a Comfortable Sleep Environment:** Make sure your bedroom is dark, quiet, and at a comfortable temperature. Invest in a supportive mattress and pillows that promote proper alignment and comfort.
- **Avoid Electronic Devices:** The blue light emitted by electronic devices can disrupt your sleep-wake cycle. Avoid using smartphones, tablets, and computers for at least an hour before bed.
- **Avoid Heavy Meals:** Eating a heavy meal close to bedtime can cause discomfort and indigestion, making it difficult to fall asleep. Opt for a light, balanced snack if you're hungry before bed.

- **Practice Relaxation Techniques:** Incorporate relaxation techniques such as meditation, gentle stretching, or progressive muscle relaxation into your bedtime routine. These techniques can help reduce stress and promote relaxation.

By establishing a bedtime routine that prioritizes relaxation and quality sleep, you can support your fertility journey and enhance your overall well-being. Remember, consistency is key, so stick to your routine as much as possible to reap the benefits.

Avoid Electronic Devices Before Bed

Avoiding electronic devices before bed is crucial for ensuring a good night's sleep and promoting fertility. The screens of electronic devices, such as smartphones, tablets, and laptops, emit blue light that can disrupt the body's natural sleep-wake cycle, also known as the circadian rhythm. This disruption can lead to difficulties falling asleep and staying asleep, ultimately affecting the quality and duration of sleep.

Moreover, the negative effects of screens on sleep can also impact fertility. Research has shown that inadequate sleep or poor sleep quality can interfere with reproductive hormones and menstrual cycles, potentially affecting ovulation and fertility. Therefore, it is important to minimize exposure to electronic devices before bed to optimize both sleep and fertility.

To minimize exposure to screens before bed, consider implementing the following strategies:

- Establish a bedtime routine that does not involve electronic devices. Engage in relaxing activities such as reading a book, taking a warm bath, or practicing gentle stretching exercises.
- Create a screen-free zone in your bedroom. Remove electronic devices from your sleeping area to eliminate the temptation of using them before bed.
- Set a specific time to disconnect from electronic devices. Aim to turn off screens at least one hour before bedtime to allow your body to prepare for sleep.
- Use blue light filters or apps that reduce the amount of blue light emitted by your devices. These filters can help minimize the impact of screens on your sleep and fertility.

By avoiding electronic devices before bed, you can improve your sleep quality and enhance your fertility. Prioritizing restful sleep and creating a screen-free environment in the evening can contribute to overall well-being and increase your chances of conceiving.

Reduce Exposure to Environmental Toxins

Reducing exposure to environmental toxins is crucial for optimizing fertility. There are various common environmental toxins that can have a negative impact on reproductive health. By identifying these toxins and taking steps to minimize exposure, individuals can improve their chances of conceiving.

Some of the common environmental toxins that can affect fertility include:

- Chemicals in household products: Certain chemicals found in everyday household products, such as cleaning agents, cosmetics, and personal care items, can disrupt hormonal balance and interfere with reproductive processes. It is important to read labels carefully and choose products that are free from harmful chemicals.
- Pesticides: Exposure to pesticides, whether through contaminated food or direct contact, has been linked to fertility problems. To minimize exposure, opt for organic produce whenever possible and wash fruits and vegetables thoroughly before consumption.

To reduce exposure to environmental toxins and promote fertility, consider the following strategies:

- Use natural and eco-friendly household products: Look for alternatives to common household products that are free from harmful chemicals. There are many environmentally friendly options available that are safe for both your health and the environment.
- Choose organic food: Opt for organic fruits, vegetables, and meats to reduce exposure to pesticides and other harmful chemicals. Organic farming practices prioritize the use of natural fertilizers and pest control methods.
- Filter your water: Install a water filtration system to remove potential toxins and contaminants from your drinking water. This can help reduce exposure to harmful substances that may affect fertility.
- Minimize exposure to air pollutants: Avoid spending extended periods of time in areas with high levels of air pollution. If possible, use air purifiers in your home to improve indoor air quality.

By being mindful of the environmental toxins that can impact fertility and taking proactive steps to minimize exposure, individuals can create a healthier and more conducive environment for conception.

Avoid Harmful Chemicals in Household Products

Avoiding harmful chemicals in household products is crucial for maintaining fertility and reproductive health. Many common household products contain chemicals that can disrupt hormonal balance and negatively impact fertility. These chemicals, known as endocrine disruptors, can mimic or interfere with the body's natural hormones, leading to fertility issues.

One of the main culprits is phthalates, which are commonly found in fragrances, plastics, and personal care products. Phthalates have been linked to decreased sperm quality and hormone imbalances in both men and women. To avoid phthalates, opt for fragrance-free products and choose natural alternatives for cleaning and personal care.

Another chemical to watch out for is bisphenol A (BPA), which is often found in plastic containers and food packaging. BPA has been associated with hormonal disruptions and reduced fertility. To minimize exposure to BPA, opt for glass or stainless steel containers for food storage and avoid microwaving food in plastic containers.

Furthermore, certain cleaning products contain chemicals like triclosan and ammonia, which can also interfere with reproductive health. These chemicals can be replaced with natural alternatives such as vinegar, baking soda, and essential oils, which are equally effective in cleaning without the harmful side effects.

It's important to read labels carefully and educate yourself about the potential dangers of chemicals in household products. Look for products that are labeled as "phthalate-free," "BPA-free," and "chemical-free." Additionally, consider making your own cleaning products using simple ingredients like vinegar, lemon juice, and baking soda.

By avoiding harmful chemicals in household products, you can protect your fertility and create a healthier environment for yourself and your family. Taking these small steps towards reducing exposure to endocrine disruptors can make a significant difference in your reproductive health and overall well-being.

Limit Exposure to Pesticides

Limit Exposure to Pesticides

Pesticides are chemicals used to control pests and weeds in agriculture and household settings. However, these chemicals have the potential to negatively impact fertility. Studies have shown that exposure to pesticides can disrupt hormone levels, interfere with reproductive processes, and even lead to infertility.

To reduce your exposure to pesticides and protect your fertility, consider the following tips:

- Choose organic produce whenever possible: Organic fruits and vegetables are grown without the use of synthetic pesticides, reducing your exposure to harmful chemicals.
- Wash fruits and vegetables thoroughly: Washing produce under running water can help remove some pesticide residues.
- Peel non-organic fruits and vegetables: Peeling can further reduce pesticide residues, although keep in mind that some nutrients may be lost in the process.
- Avoid using pesticides in your home: Opt for natural alternatives or seek professional pest control services that use safer methods.
- Be cautious with garden pesticides: If you use pesticides in your garden, follow the instructions carefully and consider using organic or natural alternatives.
- Limit exposure to treated areas: Stay away from areas where pesticides have recently been applied, and avoid contact with treated surfaces.

By taking these precautions and reducing your exposure to pesticides, you can help protect your fertility and overall reproductive health.

Stay Hydrated

Stay Hydrated

Hydration is a crucial factor when it comes to fertility. It plays a vital role in maintaining the overall health of your reproductive system. Staying hydrated ensures that your body has enough fluids to support the production of cervical mucus, which is essential for sperm to travel through the cervix and reach the egg.

Drinking an adequate amount of water also helps in optimizing the quality of your cervical mucus. When you are dehydrated, your cervical mucus tends to become thick and sticky, making it difficult for sperm to swim freely. By staying hydrated, you can promote the production of fertile cervical mucus that is thin, slippery, and favorable for sperm survival and movement.

To ensure that you are adequately hydrated, it is recommended to drink at least 8 to 10 glasses of water per day. However, the exact amount may vary depending on individual needs and activity levels. It is important to listen to your body and drink water whenever you feel thirsty.

In addition to water, you can also include other hydrating fluids in your diet, such as herbal teas, fresh fruit juices, and coconut water. These beverages not only help in maintaining hydration but also provide essential nutrients that support overall reproductive health.

Remember, staying hydrated is a simple yet effective way to boost your fertility naturally. By prioritizing your water intake, you can create a favorable environment for conception and increase your chances of getting pregnant.

Quit Smoking

Quit Smoking

Smoking has a detrimental effect on fertility, both for men and women. Research has shown that smoking can reduce the quality of sperm in men, leading to decreased fertility. In women, smoking can disrupt the delicate balance of hormones necessary for ovulation and implantation of a fertilized egg. It can also damage the fallopian tubes and increase the risk of miscarriage.

If you are trying to conceive, quitting smoking is crucial. Not only will it improve your chances of getting pregnant, but it will also have numerous other health benefits for you and your future baby. Quitting smoking can be challenging, but with the right strategies and support, it is possible.

Here are some strategies for quitting smoking:

- Set a quit date and stick to it. Having a specific date to work towards can help you stay motivated.
- Find support. Reach out to friends, family, or support groups who can provide encouragement and accountability.
- Consider nicotine replacement therapy. Products such as nicotine patches, gum, or inhalers can help reduce withdrawal symptoms.
- Explore alternative therapies. Some people find success with acupuncture, hypnosis, or other alternative treatments to aid in smoking cessation.
- Stay active and distract yourself. Engaging in physical activity can help reduce cravings, and finding activities or hobbies that keep your mind occupied can help take your focus away from smoking.

Remember, quitting smoking is not only beneficial for your fertility, but it also improves your overall health and reduces the risk of numerous diseases. Seek support, stay motivated, and take one day at a time on your journey to become smoke-free.

Seek Support to Quit Smoking

When it comes to quitting smoking, seeking support is crucial for success. There are various resources and support systems available to help individuals quit smoking and improve their fertility. These resources can provide guidance, motivation, and accountability throughout the quitting process.

One option for seeking support is joining a smoking cessation program or support group. These programs are designed specifically for individuals who want to quit smoking and provide a supportive environment where participants can share their experiences and learn from others. They often offer counseling, educational materials, and strategies for managing cravings and withdrawal symptoms.

Another valuable resource is healthcare professionals. Doctors, nurses, and other healthcare providers can offer personalized guidance and support tailored to an individual's specific needs and circumstances. They can provide information about the impact of smoking on fertility and offer strategies to quit smoking effectively. Healthcare professionals may also be able to prescribe medications or recommend other interventions to aid in the quitting process.

In addition to formal programs and healthcare professionals, there are numerous online resources available to help individuals quit smoking. Websites, forums, and mobile applications provide information, tips, and support for those looking to quit. These platforms often offer interactive tools, such as quit trackers and calculators, to monitor progress and provide motivation.

Support from friends and family members is also crucial during the quitting process. Loved ones can offer encouragement, understanding, and accountability. They can help create a smoke-free environment and provide distractions or alternative activities to replace smoking habits.

Remember, quitting smoking is not easy, but with the right support, it is possible. Whether it's through formal programs, healthcare professionals, online resources, or the support of loved ones, seeking support can greatly increase the chances of successfully quitting smoking and improving fertility.

Limit Alcohol Consumption

Limit Alcohol Consumption

Alcohol consumption has been linked to fertility problems, making it important to limit your intake if you're trying to conceive. Excessive alcohol consumption can disrupt hormone levels and interfere with reproductive processes, leading to difficulties in getting pregnant. It can also increase the risk of miscarriage and negatively impact the health of the developing fetus.

To maximize your chances of conceiving, it's recommended to follow guidelines for moderate drinking. These guidelines vary by country, but generally, it's advised to limit alcohol consumption to no more than one drink per day for women and two drinks per day for men. Keep in mind that even moderate alcohol intake can still affect fertility, so it's best to consider abstaining from alcohol altogether when trying to conceive.

Creating a supportive environment for fertility involves making conscious choices about what you consume. By limiting alcohol consumption, you're taking a proactive step towards optimizing your reproductive health and increasing your chances of conception.

Avoid Excessive Caffeine

Avoid Excessive Caffeine

Caffeine, found in coffee, tea, soda, and chocolate, is a stimulant that can have negative effects on fertility. While moderate caffeine consumption is generally considered safe, excessive intake can interfere with reproductive health. Studies have shown that high levels of caffeine can disrupt hormone levels and impair fertility in both men and women.

When it comes to caffeine and fertility, it's important to find a balance. The recommended limit for caffeine consumption is typically around 200-300 milligrams per day, which is roughly equivalent to one or two cups of coffee. However, it's important to note that caffeine content can vary depending on the type of beverage or food consumed.

To help you keep track of your caffeine intake, here is a table showing the approximate caffeine content in common sources:

Beverage/Food	Caffeine Content (mg)
Coffee (8 oz)	95-165
Black Tea (8 oz)	25-48
Green Tea (8 oz)	25-29
Soda (12 oz)	30-55
Dark Chocolate (1 oz)	12-30

It's important to note that caffeine sensitivity can vary from person to person, so it's best to listen to your body and adjust your caffeine intake accordingly. If you're trying to conceive, it may be wise to limit your caffeine consumption to ensure optimal fertility.

In addition to the potential effects on fertility, excessive caffeine intake can also have other negative impacts on overall health, such as disrupted sleep patterns and increased anxiety. Therefore, it's important to be mindful of your caffeine consumption and make informed choices for your reproductive well-being.

Track Your Menstrual Cycle

The menstrual cycle plays a crucial role in a woman's fertility. Understanding and tracking your menstrual cycle can greatly optimize your chances of conceiving. By monitoring the various phases of your cycle, you can identify the most fertile days and time intercourse accordingly.

One effective method for tracking your menstrual cycle is through the use of ovulation prediction kits. These kits detect the surge in luteinizing hormone (LH) that occurs just before ovulation. By testing your urine with the kit, you can pinpoint the most fertile days of your cycle and plan intercourse accordingly.

Another method for tracking your menstrual cycle is by monitoring your basal body temperature (BBT). This involves taking your temperature every morning before getting out of bed. A slight increase in BBT indicates that ovulation has occurred. By charting your BBT over several months, you can identify patterns and predict when ovulation is likely to occur in future cycles.

Tracking your menstrual cycle not only helps optimize fertility but also provides valuable insights into your reproductive health. It can help identify irregularities or potential issues that may need medical attention. By understanding your menstrual cycle, you can take proactive steps towards achieving your goal of conception.

Use Ovulation Prediction Kits

Using ovulation prediction kits can greatly assist in determining the most fertile days of your menstrual cycle. These kits work by detecting the surge in luteinizing hormone (LH) that occurs right before ovulation. By tracking this hormone, you can pinpoint the optimal time for conception.

Ovulation prediction kits are easy to use and typically involve collecting a urine sample and testing it with the provided strip or device. The kit will indicate whether or not the LH surge has occurred, indicating that ovulation is imminent. This allows you to plan intercourse accordingly, increasing your chances of successful conception.

It's important to note that ovulation prediction kits are most effective for women with regular menstrual cycles. If your cycle is irregular, it may be more challenging to accurately predict ovulation using these kits alone. In such cases, it may be helpful to track additional signs of ovulation, such as changes in cervical mucus or basal body temperature.

By incorporating ovulation prediction kits into your fertility journey, you can take a proactive approach to maximizing your chances of conceiving. These kits provide valuable information about your hormonal patterns, allowing you to make informed decisions about timing intercourse and optimizing fertility.

Monitor Basal Body Temperature

Monitor Basal Body Temperature

When it comes to tracking ovulation and fertility, monitoring basal body temperature (BBT) can be a valuable tool. Basal body temperature refers to your body's temperature at rest, and it can provide important insights into your menstrual cycle.

During the first half of your menstrual cycle, known as the follicular phase, your BBT is typically lower. However, after ovulation occurs, there is a slight increase in BBT due to the release of the hormone progesterone. This rise in temperature can indicate that ovulation has taken place.

To accurately monitor your basal body temperature, it is important to take your temperature at the same time every morning before getting out of bed. This consistency ensures accurate readings. You can use a basal body thermometer, which is more sensitive and precise than a regular thermometer.

It is recommended to keep a record of your daily temperatures on a chart or in a fertility tracking app. This will help you identify patterns and determine when ovulation is likely to occur in your cycle. By tracking your BBT over several cycles, you can gain a better understanding of your unique fertility patterns.

It's important to note that BBT alone cannot predict the exact day of ovulation, as the temperature rise occurs after ovulation. However, when combined with other fertility tracking methods such as cervical mucus monitoring and ovulation prediction kits, monitoring basal body temperature can provide valuable information for maximizing your chances of conception.

Consider Herbal Supplements

Consider Herbal Supplements

When it comes to enhancing fertility, certain herbal supplements have shown potential benefits. These supplements are derived from natural sources and are believed to support reproductive health and increase the chances of conception. While it's important to consult with a healthcare professional before incorporating any new supplements into your routine, here are some herbal options that have been associated with fertility enhancement:

- Vitex (Chasteberry): This herb is known for its ability to regulate hormone levels and promote a healthy menstrual cycle. It may help balance estrogen and progesterone levels, leading to improved fertility.
- Maca Root: Maca is a root vegetable that has been used for centuries to enhance fertility. It is believed to support hormonal balance and increase libido, potentially improving the chances of conception.
- Raspberry Leaf: Raspberry leaf is often used to strengthen the uterus and prepare it for pregnancy. It is rich in vitamins and minerals that support reproductive health.
- Dong Quai: Dong Quai is an herb commonly used in traditional Chinese medicine to promote fertility. It is believed to regulate hormone levels and improve blood flow to the reproductive organs.

It's important to note that while herbal supplements can offer potential benefits, they should be used with caution and under the guidance of a healthcare professional. Some herbs may interact with medications or have contraindications for certain medical conditions. Therefore, it's crucial to seek professional advice before incorporating herbal supplements into your fertility journey.

Consult with a Healthcare Professional

When considering herbal supplements for fertility enhancement, it is crucial to consult with a healthcare professional. While herbal remedies may offer potential benefits, it is essential to seek professional advice before incorporating them into your fertility journey.

A healthcare professional, such as a doctor or a fertility specialist, can provide valuable guidance and ensure that the supplements you are considering are safe and appropriate for your specific situation. They can assess your medical history, evaluate any underlying conditions, and determine if herbal supplements are a suitable option for you.

Additionally, healthcare professionals have extensive knowledge and experience in the field of fertility. They can provide expert advice on the most effective supplements, dosages, and potential interactions with any medications you may be taking. They can also monitor your progress and make adjustments to your treatment plan if necessary.

Remember, herbal supplements are not regulated in the same way as prescription medications, and their safety and effectiveness may vary. By consulting with a healthcare professional, you can make informed decisions and ensure that you are taking the right steps to enhance your fertility safely and effectively.

Have Regular Sexual Intercourse

Having regular sexual intercourse is of utmost importance when it comes to maximizing fertility. It is a key factor in increasing the chances of conception and achieving pregnancy. When a couple engages in regular sexual activity, especially during the woman's fertile window, the likelihood of sperm meeting the egg is significantly higher.

Regular intercourse ensures that there is a constant supply of fresh and healthy sperm in the reproductive system. Sperm can survive in the female reproductive tract for up to five days, so having sex every two to three days throughout the menstrual cycle can increase the chances of sperm being present during ovulation.

It's important to understand and track the woman's menstrual cycle to determine the most fertile days. Ovulation prediction kits can be used to identify the surge in luteinizing hormone (LH) that occurs before ovulation. This surge indicates that ovulation is about to occur, and it's the ideal time to have intercourse. Monitoring basal body temperature can also help pinpoint the timing of ovulation.

While the focus may be on increasing fertility, it's essential to remember to enjoy the process. Trying to conceive can sometimes become stressful, but maintaining a positive mindset and enjoying the journey towards conception can have a positive impact on both physical and emotional well-being. Stress can interfere with fertility, so finding ways to relax and connect with your partner can be beneficial.

In conclusion, regular sexual intercourse is vital for maximizing fertility. Understanding the menstrual cycle, timing intercourse with ovulation, and maintaining a positive mindset are key factors in increasing the chances of conception. Remember to enjoy the process and seek support if needed. With patience and persistence, you can increase your chances of achieving a successful pregnancy.

Timing Intercourse with Ovulation

When it comes to maximizing your chances of conception, timing is everything. Understanding your ovulation cycle is crucial in determining the best time to have intercourse for optimal fertility. Ovulation is the process in which a mature egg is released from the ovary, ready to be fertilized by sperm.

There are several methods you can use to track your ovulation and time intercourse accordingly. One effective method is using ovulation prediction kits, also known as OPKs. These kits detect the surge in luteinizing hormone (LH) that occurs approximately 24 to 36 hours before ovulation. By monitoring the levels of LH in your urine, OPKs can help you pinpoint the most fertile days of your cycle.

Another method is monitoring your basal body temperature (BBT). Your BBT is your body's lowest resting temperature, which slightly increases after ovulation due to the release of progesterone. By charting your BBT daily, you can identify the slight rise that indicates ovulation has occurred. This can help you time intercourse during your most fertile days.

It's important to note that sperm can survive in the female reproductive tract for up to five days, while the egg is only viable for about 24 hours after ovulation. Therefore, it's recommended to have intercourse in the days leading up to ovulation to increase the chances of sperm being present when the egg is released.

Remember, trying to conceive should be a joyful and intimate experience. While timing intercourse with ovulation is important, it's equally important to maintain a positive mindset and enjoy the journey towards conception. Stress and pressure can negatively impact fertility, so try to relax and let nature take its course.

Enjoy the Process

The journey towards conception can be filled with ups and downs, and it's important to maintain a positive mindset throughout. While it's natural to feel anxious or impatient, stressing over the process can actually hinder fertility. When you are constantly focused on the end result, it can create unnecessary pressure and tension.

Instead, try to shift your focus to enjoying the journey itself. Embrace the special moments with your partner, nurture your relationship, and find joy in the process of trying to conceive. Remember, conception is a beautiful and intimate experience that can bring you closer together.

Take time to celebrate small victories along the way, such as tracking your menstrual cycle accurately or making positive lifestyle changes. Surround yourself with a support system of loved ones who can provide encouragement and understanding. By maintaining a positive mindset, you can reduce stress levels and create a more conducive environment for conception.

It's important to remember that the journey towards conception is unique for every couple. While it may take longer for some, it's essential to stay patient and trust in the process. Enjoy the moments of intimacy and connection with your partner, and cherish the anticipation and excitement that comes with trying to conceive.

Ultimately, the journey towards conception should be seen as a beautiful chapter in your life, filled with hope and love. Embrace the process, stay positive, and trust that your time will come.

Frequently Asked Questions

- **Q: How can nutrition impact fertility?**

  A: Nutrition plays a crucial role in fertility as certain nutrients are essential for reproductive health. A well-balanced diet rich in fruits, vegetables, whole grains, and lean proteins can provide the necessary vitamins and minerals to support fertility.

- **Q: Can stress affect fertility?**

  A: Yes, high levels of stress can negatively impact fertility. Stress can disrupt hormonal balance and interfere with the ovulation process. It is important to find effective stress reduction techniques and incorporate them into your daily routine.

- **Q: How does exercise affect fertility?**

  A: Regular exercise has been shown to improve fertility by promoting hormonal balance, reducing stress, and maintaining a healthy weight. Moderate exercise, such as brisk walking or swimming, is recommended for optimal fertility.

- **Q: Does weight play a role in fertility?**

  A: Yes, both extreme weight loss and obesity can negatively impact fertility. It is important to maintain a healthy weight as it can affect hormone production and ovulation. Consulting with a healthcare professional can provide guidance on achieving a healthy weight for fertility.

- **Q: How does sleep affect fertility?**

  A: Sufficient sleep is essential for reproductive health. Poor sleep quality and inadequate sleep duration can disrupt hormone production and affect fertility. Establishing a bedtime routine and minimizing exposure to electronic devices before bed can help improve sleep and fertility.

- **Q: Are environmental toxins harmful to fertility?**

  A: Yes, exposure to certain environmental toxins can impact fertility. Harmful chemicals in household products and pesticides can disrupt hormonal balance and affect reproductive health. Minimizing exposure to these toxins is recommended for optimizing fertility.

- **Q: Is quitting smoking important for fertility?**

  A: Yes, smoking can significantly decrease fertility in both men and women. Quitting smoking is crucial for improving reproductive health and increasing the chances of conception. Seeking support from resources and support systems can aid in the quitting process.

- **Q: How does alcohol consumption affect fertility?**

  A: Excessive alcohol consumption can negatively impact fertility. It is advisable to limit alcohol intake to moderate levels or avoid it altogether when trying to conceive. Following guidelines for moderate drinking can help maintain reproductive health.

- **Q: Can caffeine affect fertility?**

  A: Yes, excessive caffeine intake has been associated with fertility problems. It is recommended to limit caffeine consumption to moderate levels, as high caffeine intake can interfere with hormone production and affect fertility.

- **Q: How can tracking the menstrual cycle help with fertility?**

  A: Understanding your menstrual cycle is vital for optimizing fertility. Tracking ovulation through methods such as ovulation prediction kits and monitoring basal body temperature can help identify the most fertile days of the cycle and increase the chances of conception.

- **Q: Are herbal supplements beneficial for fertility?**

A: Certain herbal supplements may have potential benefits for enhancing fertility. However, it is important to consult with a healthcare professional before taking any herbal supplements to ensure safety and effectiveness.

- **Q: How does regular sexual intercourse impact fertility?**

A: Regular sexual intercourse throughout the menstrual cycle increases the chances of conception. It is recommended to time intercourse with ovulation to maximize fertility. It is also important to maintain a positive mindset and enjoy the process of trying to conceive.

Have Questions / Comments?

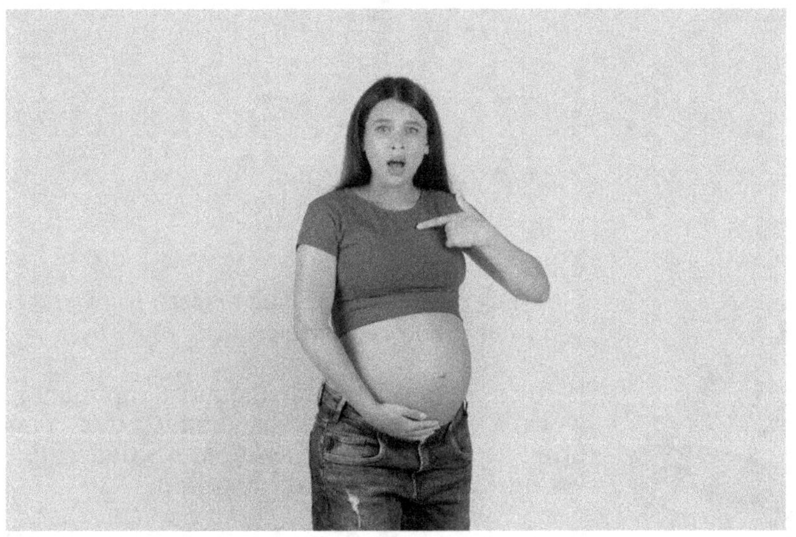

This book was designed to cover as much info as possible but I know I have probably missed something, or some new amazing discovery that has just come out.

If you notice something missing or have a question that I failed to answer, please get in touch and let me know. If I can, I will email you an answer and also update the book so others can also benefit from it.

Thanks For Being Awesome :)

Submit Your Questions / Comments At:
Get In Touch Babydreamers.net

Get How To Be A Super Mom 100% FREE

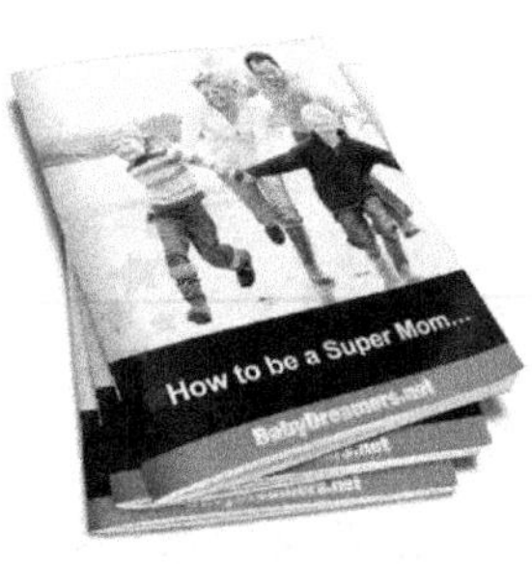

For being one of our amazing readers, we would love to offer you another book we have created, 100% free.

Being a mom is probably the most important job in the world – we've all heard that, and it's true. You're bringing up the next generation of wonderful, intelligent, loving, creative, responsible people.

We all want to be Super Mom and to be everything and do everything, but it this possible?

Being a Super Mom is possible, but you have to learn how to empower yourself to be the kind of Super Mom that you feel you need to be, keeping in mind that the title Super Mom doesn't mean the same thing to everyone.

<u>Get How to be a Super Mom For Free</u>